BODYBUILDING

The Formula of Hypertrophy - Optimize Training

(The Complete Blueprint to Building Muscle With Weight Lifting)

Richard Cortez

Published By **Richard Cortez**

Richard Cortez

Bodybuilding: The Formula of Hypertrophy - Optimize Training (The Complete Blueprint to Building Muscle With Weight Lifting)

ISBN 978-1-77485-442-6

Legal & Disclaimer

The information contained in this book is not designed to replace or take the place of any form of medicine or professional medical advice. The information in this book has been provided for educational and entertainment purposes only.

The information contained in this book has been compiled from sources deemed reliable, and it is accurate to the best of the Author's knowledge; however, the Author cannot guarantee its accuracy and validity and cannot be held liable for any errors or omissions. Changes are periodically made to this book. You must consult your doctor or get professional medical advice before using any of the suggested remedies, techniques, or information in this book.

Upon using the information contained in this book, you agree to hold harmless the Author from and against any damages, costs, and expenses, including any legal fees potentially resulting from the application of any of the information provided by this guide. This disclaimer applies to any damages or injury caused by the use and application, whether directly or indirectly, of any advice or information presented, whether for breach of contract, tort, negligence, personal injury, criminal intent, or under any other cause of action.

You agree to accept all risks of using the information presented inside this book. You need to consult a professional medical practitioner in order to ensure you are both able and healthy enough to participate in this program.

TABLE OF CONTENTS

Introduction

I know that you've spent hours scrolling through the multitude of muscle-training supplements and methods available. But this one is different. This book is for those people who get squeamish when they see bizarre-colored drinks from Whole Foods. This book is designed for people who are not willing to wear tshirts too small to showoff their muscles. This book will appeal to people who can't afford to spend hundreds a month at the GNC just for the "latest in supplements." It also won't be recommended for anyone contemplating using dangerous hormone/steroid combos. This book will not make you look like Ahnold, or any of those body-builders. This book outlines proven steps and strategies to increase your body's capacity to build lean muscles and burn fat. The Five Color Supps are a safe, effective, and affordable way to get fit and healthy. Intrigued? So were we! Follow these steps to develop your body muscles.

Chapter 1: Why Should A Female Bodybuilder Work?

A lot of women are interested in fitness and have many concerns. There are many reasons you should become a female bodybuilder. Ob you are competing or looking for a tough body, fitness is vital to your mental and physical health. Here are some of the reasons you should be training to become female bodybuilder.

Reason #1 - Increasing muscle mass can lead you to burning more fat. Studies have shown that each pound of muscle your body gains can result in a 35-50% increase in calories burned per day. Doing so will help increase your body's metabolic rate, thereby increasing your lean muscle mass. Even if your couch is all you have, your body will still be burning calories.

Reason #2 - Building muscle is the best way to increase strength. Many women worry that by lifting heavy they will bulk up. As we'll see, it is nearly impossible because of the biology inherent in women's bodies. Short story: Strength training alone is enough to help women achieve muscle tone, definition, and strength.

Third Reason: Training not only will you build strength but it will make you feel better overall. This will allow you to become less dependent on other people. If you are required to lift laundry, grocery, or children's groceries, all you will require is yourself and your muscles. This is just another perk that comes with being a strong and independent woman bodybuilder.

Reason #4 - Bodybuilding can help you improve your health. Women who lift weights are known to have a lower risk of developing diabetes. Research shows that weight training can help the body handle sugar more effectively by increasing glucose utilization. You'll look amazing on the inside and outside!

Reason #5 Weight training is also a great way to reduce the risk of developing arthritis, back pain or other injuries. Bodybuilding helps build strong connective tissues and enhances joint stability. You will also be able to keep your muscles strong and flexible with weight training. It's a great way of preventing injuries and keeping your muscles toned.

Reason #6. Weight training can help lower your chances of getting heart disease. Exercise has been proven to lower the likelihood of obesity, high blood sugar and high cholesterol among women who have participated in physical activity.

Reason #7. Bodybuilding is essential for your mental and physical health. Studies have shown that weight training can reduce mental tension and fatigue. This activity will increase your mood and release endorphins. Exercise can help with anxiety, depression, stress reduction, and other issues like stress management. Exercise can make you feel happier and will help you get out of bed each morning.

Every positive aspect has its cons. We aren't here to tell bodybuilding that it is a wonderful sport. There is always something wrong. Here are some reasons not to get involved in bodybuilding.

Reason #1. Although bodybuilding can lower your chances of getting an accident, there is always the risk of getting hurt. This is most common when someone lifts a large amount of weight. Injuries can occur when your body is put under strain by lifting too heavy. This is why it is important to vary how heavy you lift and how often you exercise. Lower back and shoulder injuries are the most common among bodybuilders. There are correct lifting techniques that can keep you safe from injury.

Reason #2. If you do intend on lifting weights you should keep cardio in your mind. Cardio will be more beneficial for you if your muscle mass is greater than your cardio. Because your body needs strong cardio systems to pump blood around your system, this is important. Some bodybuilders may skip cardio, which can cause damage to the heart. To protect your heart health, weight lifting and cardio must be done in tandem.

Reason #3. Bodybuilders need to have a regular cardio workout routine. Many bodybuilders have lost their lives due to torn Aortas. Heavy lifting can cause high blood pressure. You will need a strong cardiosystem to manage the stress. To determine if your body can handle heavy lifting, it is worth getting screened. If your body is not ready for weight lifting, it's worth starting off lighter and working your way up.

Reason #4. The "con" I am going to list last will be different for each person. Some bodybuilders resort to severe diets to gain the competitive edge. Sometimes, this involves deliberately dehydrating yourself or eating excessive amounts of protein. There are healthy options to ensure your body is not damaged while still achieving the results you want. There's no reason to take steroids or use chemical shortcuts in order to get the results you want faster. These elements can lead liver damage, high blood pressure, heart disease, anxiety, depression, and heart disease.

As you can see there are many perks to starting weight training. It is about how to navigate it so it is safe. In the next chapter we will discuss some nutrition tips for female bodybuilders to help take your game higher.

Chapter 2: Bodybuilding Basics

Bodybuilding is an ancient way to enhance your muscles. It involves working out and following diets that increase muscle mass. It's often done for recreational purposes or personal growth. Bodybuilding gained popularity over time as a competitive sports activity. Bodybuilding is also known by the term "hard gaining", which is a program for people who don't intend to gain muscle mass.

This activity is frequently confused with weight training. Bodybuilding emphasizes improving the appearance of your muscles by shaping and increasing muscle mass. This is not about strength and agility.

It is unlikely that women who are bodybuilding will have a bigger, more muscular body. The hormone testosterone is responsible to the bulk that male bodybuilders display. This hormone is stimulated in the gym by men who have high testosterone levels. The more testosterone, the more muscle is created. There is much less testosterone in the body for women. The normal testosterone levels in men are approximately 200-1200 ng/dl. It is between 200 and 1200 ng/dl for men. For women, it is only around 15 to 70% ng/dl. On average testosterone levels in men are 16.47x greater than in women. The difference in muscle mass between men and women is why the females gain less muscle. Bodybuilding won't give you adequate muscle growth unless it is supplemented with testosterone (steroids or other testosterone sources).

Bodybuilding requires both exercise and a healthy diet. You need to eat more often and plan your meals carefully in order for muscle gain. It is important to try different workouts so that your body can benefit from them all. You will find the most enjoyable workouts because they are entertaining and your motivation is high.

How to get into bodybuilding

Start training for bodybuilding four days a week for women who want to tone and build muscle. Allow enough time for rest and training. The muscles require a 72-hour break after high volume, high intensity workouts. Split the workouts up into separate days. One day is for leg, back, shoulder, and bicep exercises, with another for chest or shoulder workouts.

Each session should have a high level of intensity and volume. Each exercise should always be done in three sets. Each set should contain 6-12 repetitions. Each set can have only 12 repetitions. Allow 30 to 90 seconds for relaxation between sets. This is what you should do for the first few weeks. Sets can be increased to 4-6 for each type after that.

You should choose exercises that target larger muscle areas first, when you're choosing from many options. Exercise the chest, shoulder and arm muscles first before working the arms. Before exercising your legs and calves you need to work the back muscles, the buttocks and the buttocks.

The most important thing in bodybuilding is to select the right weights. Start with lighter and work your way up. For more lean body mass, challenge your muscles.

Chapter 3: Understanding Your Body

Muscle building and losing weight is not as easy as lifting weights. This change in lifestyle requires a complete overhaul. You need to make lifestyle changes, such as changing your work hours, eating habits, sleeping patterns, and mental outlook. To achieve all these, you must have the necessary knowledge about your body's workings.

Understanding Muscles

All people know that muscles allow your body to walk, move, eat and perform any other motor function. Muscles are there to keep you afloat. Without them, vital organs like your heart and lungs could not function. Looking good is one reason that many people - male and female - love being lean.

Also, bodybuilding will not only improve your appearance but also make you more attractive. These are perks, not a way to be more attractive or look better. When you exercise to increase muscle mass, your metabolism works faster to eliminate toxins and burn excess fat.

Strength training can have a positive impact on your nervous system as well as your cardiovascular and respiratory systems. It also improves circulation and oxygen supply to your body. Training reduces your risk of suffering from bone-related injuries in the future.

What is your body type

It might seem strange that some people build muscles faster than others, even though it may seem unfair. This is partly due to genes that influence metabolism and body frame. Today's world of exercise and fitness should teach you about the following body types.

Ectomorph: The endomorph refers to the "skinny", slimmest body type. People who fall under this category have shorter joints, narrower hips, longer limbs, which contributes greatly to their slim appearance. They tend to have flat chests with low muscle mass. Their fast metabolism makes it difficult for them not to gain weight, or even build muscle.

Endomorphs - Although they gain muscles faster than ectomorphs but gain fat faster than most other body types, endomorphs tend to be more muscular than ectomorphs. They have shorter arms and legs, as well as a wider body. Their figure is often soft around the neck and upper body. They also have a slower metabolism than the other two body types making it difficult to lose excess fat.

Mesomorph- The last of the body types, the mesomorph, is the naturally athletic and well-looking one. They have a slimmer waistline and more joints than endomorphs. But they have larger shoulders and clavicles that ectomorphs. They can rapidly build muscle mass and quickly lose excess fat through regular exercise.

While the mesomorph might be the most suitable body type to bodybuild, it's important to keep in mind the benefits of endomorphs. Endomorphs gain mass quickly, which allows the individual early to see the results of muscle-building. Ectomorphs, on other hand, are able to maintain a desirable body-to-fat ratio and can remain slim. These are good to have in your routine. But it's more important to understand the strengths of these body types.

Note that you can combine a body type with a mesomorph one, but not all three. Although your body type can be easily identified, keep in mind that your lifestyle and current habits will impact how your appearance. Use the following tests to find out your body type.

**Twist your middle finger and thumb around the other side of your wrist.

#The tip between your thumb and middle finger meets - Endomorph/Mesomorph

#The tip of your middle finger may overlap with your thumb - Mesomorph/Ectomorph

#Your fingers never touch - Endomorph

**If standing straight:

#Your shoulders are slightly higher than your hips.

#Your hips are larger than your shoulders. Endomorph

**If weight changes have occurred in the recent past:

#Endometromorphs: You find it difficult to maintain your weight.

#Ectomorphs can have a lot of food and not gain weight.

#Mesomorphs don't struggle to lose or gain weight.

Your doctor is a good option if you're trying to figure out your body type. Your personalized training program might require a different approach depending o your body type. These points will be included in any of the strategies or activities that are available.

Your Personalized Fitness Plan

Everybody can be fit and toned, no matter their body type. This book will concentrate on two things that you can do at your own home: exercise and nutrition. These are your key components for your personalized fitness plan.

Going to the gym and using specialized tools like everyone else is good. However, that's something you will need to do in the future. It is best to get your life in order now and start planning your individual fitness plan.

Chapter 4: Getting Started

Everything in life has a beginning point. Bodybuilding, like all things, starts from the ground floor. You can't begin from the bottom or the middle. Lifting and exercising should be done gradually. However, there are many people who start lifting weights from the very beginning. This can cause muscle torment and may result in a loss of strength for a few months.

As a beginner in this sport, you need to have a plan. You can make the biggest mistake in this area by trying to do too much at once. Expert bodybuilders will tell you to slow down and stick to a plan. Even though you might be unsure of how to put together a plan, this article will show you the steps. It may take longer but the results you'll get will be more durable and will make you look better.

1. Get Clear on Your Goal

Everybody starts bodybuilding for a variety of reasons. It is vital to decide which one is you. This will allow you to plan your time and schedule. It could be building muscle, gaining weight, losing weight and getting into shape. You might even want to become a model or start professional bodybuilding. What is your goal? It does not matter if you are a beginner or an expert female bodybuilder, knowing your goals will help you achieve them and motivate you to do so.

2. Find a Gym

For beginners, it is best to search in your local area for the right gym. It's even better if the nearest gym is within walking distance. There will be fewer reasons not to go if it's close. Don't forget about the atmosphere. It is crucial to your success. It will help you focus more which will lead to better results.

One thing you can decide to do is: For beginners, you have the option to work with a personal training coach. Or, you can choose to join a gym that has many bodybuilders.

3. Find a partner

Every sport has its unique challenges. Bodybuilding is no exception. It is possible to make everything seem easier with the right support and motivation. However, 90% of bodybuilders couldn't reach their goals. They didn't have the motivation or support that every beginner needs.

The goal can only be achieved by 10%. Just think about it. Would a female beginner[5] be able to succeed without support, motivation, or help? But, not everyone can afford a personal training session.

Partnering with a trainer is the best thing. This could be a family member, friend, or someone who shares your goal. Your partner will be there to support and motivate you as you work towards your goal.

4. Get Support

It is important to have some guidance as a beginner. Many gyms provide personal trainers who will assist you in any way possible. For example, he can give you advice about what foods and where to focus your energy.

Talk to your doctor, and ask him for advice on your diet. This is especially true for female bodybuilders who need a particular diet.

5. Keep track

It is important, as well as motivating, to keep track and record the progress that has been made. If there are no records of your past progress you won't be in a position to beat them. You can keep a record of your progress in either a notebook or an app for the phone. You should also take photographs of yourself in order to track your progress. One month's worth of pictures can help you see the progress you are making.

6. Don't Lose Heart

You won't be able to see much improvement in one or two months. Don't give up. Everyone is different, which means you shouldn't compare yourself to others. You must keep your head straight. Don't lose your enthusiasm and continue to work hard. If you are willing to work hard, you'll begin to see the difference.

7. Bodybuilding Knowledge

Learn everything you can about bodybuilding. Learn how vitamins and minerals can help you become more fit and get more energy. The book covers all of these subjects, but it's worth reading more to get even more information and understanding the details.

It is also an excellent idea to have your idol. Learn from him/her how he/she got started in bodybuilding, then follow his/her lead.

8. Learn about important muscle groups[6]

Bodybuilders may be part artist, part athlete. A bodybuilder is like a sculptor who uses clay for shaping things. You can make bodybuilding a success by planning out your goals. The body shape will be clearer and you'll know where to focus your efforts. You need to learn the anatomy of your body, how you can work on them, and what important muscle groups.

9. Sleep

Your training is only as good as your sleep. Good sleep will allow your body to recover faster after hard training. Not only will you feel more energized and healthy, but your mind will be clearer which will make it easier to remain motivated every day.

10. Get Organized

There are so many responsibilities in modern life that it can be hard to make time for yourself. However, if you organize your time well, you'll be able to do so. It is important to plan everything, from when your wake up until when you go to bed. It will make it easy to prepare a breakfast that will give you energy. You can also cook a delicious lunch. Your training is also important. Once you know what your day looks like, you can plan your diet or exercise program to achieve your goals. The next step is to decide what day and what kind of food you'll eat. A great organization is essential for success.

Chapter 5: Mindset Focus on The Lift

It's good that you got to your scheduled workout on time. Your laces are tied up and your heart is jogging in the rhythm you set up before the bar/handle/rope/dumbbell meet. Although your body is ready to go, it is crucial to tune in to the same frequency with your mind before you begin the warm-up. As discussed in Chapter 1, having a relaxed and focused mindset will put you at an advantage. Although it sounds complicated, it's not. It is easy to do if one is determined and does it regularly.

Many know this feeling and how valuable it is. It will become a way of life for them all. They become the person they want to be in every other endeavor. A good mental attitude will first give you safety. It will ensure that all of your positive energy flows proportionately through the blood vessels. Once that is accomplished, your focus will need to be strong enough to balance your loose thoughts.

There are many things that can distract you. Some are pretty tempting, such your favorite song. Or the song you dislike, a person who talks too loud, an addict in a gym or a person who is just plain boring. You need to discover what it is that gives you the green light. It can't be controlled if there is an empty gym.

Here is where your Mindset (determination) and focus (clear goal vision) take over. You are here for you, to feel better, and to look as good as your natural body allows. This isn't easy. You need to be willing to work hard and give your all at every training session. Now let's say you felt like you were there after the warmup. You feel comfortable and confident. Remember that you are what you think. If you are constantly bombarding your brain with negativism, it will eventually explode. This is often when you least expect it. Your body needs to be nourished like an all-inclusive dessert.

First Workset

Take the weight off and place yourself in that starting position. Be ready to pull or push, and make sure your grip remains tight. Keep inhaling and keep going. Do not let your attention wander away while you execute a move. You are still fresh from the warm up session, so you should be at the beginning point of your exercise routine. Make sure to use the mirror as often as possible. Mirrors tell you how gorgeous you are. They can also act as advisors and your personal assistants. Think about how you move and what you look like. Pay attention to the muscles of the working group. "The more that you give, the more you receive" back from them. Mirroring is not possible. You must focus on your joints, breathing, and move to the rhythm.

Sets for the Middle-Range

Your second, th, and fourth sets (or even more depending on which type of program you have) should all be very hard-pressing. What does all this mean? This means that your attention must be focused and maintained at all times. As if this is the last thing you should do, breathe deeply into your muscles. Speed is the enemy. Pros have this down pat. Chapter 5 will explain it all, and we'll touch on the Timing Agenda in Chapter 5. You should already feel your working muscle groups on fire. Another excellent tip. This tells you that you are not just on the right path, but also that your muscles are being activated to keep them attached for longer.

The Last Repeal Set

The last set differs from others slightly. The set includes all the ingredients but requires extra concentration. Your last set may not be as heavy or light depending on your program. However, you shouldn't let the happiness go yet. The so-called Drop-down Sets can sometimes make it harder for a person to do the job and get the job done. This is a major alarm. The tension causes more muscle fiber to be torn, leading to greater gains during the recovery phase. For those of you who aren't so heavy-handed critics, yes, drop-down set contains more repetitions. This allows for more muscle blood pumps/rip goals. It helps to achieve the required result because it also puts the muscle fiber under tensions.

The real question here is, are your standards of behavior respected when you bulk up?

Chapter 6: Creating a New Image for You

As you all know, change happens naturally. No matter how much you try, your body will adapt. But progress is not always easy. It's not easy to make significant progress. It takes sweat, dedication and hard work to achieve this goal. Even if the goal is to build a healthy body, feel motivated to make improvements and become stronger, there will be times when you fall short. You'll miss your workouts and lose track of your diet. Consistency will be the key to building a great physique. You can build consistency by creating long-lasting habits. Those habits will form your identity, your new YOU. You'll start to believe different things about yourself. You can make changes to your beliefs. Everyone can do it.

It is important to make a conscious decision about what you want. Be small and don't let the enormity of your goal overwhelm you. Do not think about the end. Focus on the steps, then you can get used to the process.

Here's how you can get there. Start working out consistently if you want mental and physical strength. You will see a difference in your life if you take baby steps.

What is the difference? Based on my experience, success is a combination of being motivated and showing up. It is important to always be there whether you're at the gym, running, lifting weights or sweating to achieve your goals. This lack of consistency is the main reason why most people fail in their daily lives. They haven't made this a daily routine.

Let me now give you some tips. A great way to build muscle is to work out regularly. Even if you dont notice any changes, believe me, they are coming. Be patient and lift harder than ever before. Being a champion requires you to do the hard work, train when you feel it is difficult, and lift more weight even when you are unable. If this is something that you value, you'll do what you must do. Because your priorities should be higher priority than your wants and desires. Champions know what is essential and are prepared to work tirelessly to achieve their goals. They don't always stick to the goals they set or may even abandon them altogether. They let life dictate their actions.

Another great advice I can give is this: Don't depend on motivation to build your body of dreams. Motivation doesn't last long. What will last is your habits, the system youve made for daily tasks. It is important to learn to be disciplined and to adhere to a schedule. This is the only path to being stronger, leaner, and in the best shape possible. This is what separates a true champion from a mediocre person.

Chapter 7: Chest Pecs Tits

This is the sacred grail of muscle group. A strong chest is an indicator of strength and power. It is not easy for everyone.

Growing up football-playing, I have always longed to have a big chest. As we all know defense wins games, I did everything possible to increase my size. I would work on my bench pressing every day while I stayed in the gym. It paid off, with persistence and patience. I'm not the most powerful man in the universe, but I have my moments.

It's all in the angles. Even though you may believe that the three exercises are identical, they each have a unique contribution. You have to approach it from multiple angles if you want it to be effective. (This was her point).

First, and most importantly, the highly coveted bench press. It is the star of any gym. When men have pissing matches, it is quite common to see the bench press. Mentally and physically, you will be put to the test by the bench.

You are lying on the bench with your feet firmly planted on ground. Your hands are gripping the rough bars and your back is strong and firm. You take deep inhale and exhale, and your mind wanders to that dark, mysterious place. You take the bar off the rack, and it's now time to go. The bar is you and one person must lose. You gradually lower it, keeping the dense weight in check as it nears your chest. You have now reached the halfway point. Now you want to push your chest out and squeeze your elbows into the ground. Your feet push against the ground while you push yourself away. It rises. The amazing sight of all that lifting weight back up and locking your arm. You did it. You took it down. It's almost equivalent to sacking a QB.

If you stay with it, the flat benches will deliver results. As I stated earlier, I am not a fan of 3 sets of 10, but I do believe that the flat bench can be a great tool. I love sets and sets. Limit your maxing out to once a month. If that happens, you should stick with more reps. My regular chest day usually sees me doing about 10 sets. They range in difficulty from 10 to 20, depending on how many reps I am doing. I go up and down.

It's best to start with something light. A light weight is not necessary, but enough to work your muscles and get your blood pumping. Continue to increase in increments. But everyone is different. I usually do approximately 25 lb increments.

Perform a few sets until you're pushing around 75% of maximum. Next, increase the weight of each set as you lower your weight. While 15 sets are fine, you should listen to your body. You should push yourself, not break you.

Bench Press:

Next, you'll want to do some kind of fly. When it comes my chest, I like to alternate between pushing motions with fly motions. It's a good way to give my shoulders & tris some rest between exercises.

Some may disagree with my opinion, and I don't care if they do. However, you should not be too heavy on flyes. Do you really want to go overboard with flyes? If your angle isn't right, it puts a lot strain on your shoulders. Remember that everyone is unique so try to find an angle that you can feel in your pecs. Some prefer the cables higher than others, while some prefer them to be right at their shoulders. The pleasure will still go to your shoulders, but your chest should remain the main shareholder.

As I stated before, set and reps will be followed by sets and sets. Adjust the weight according to your ability and do 8 sets. You want blood to your muscles in order for them to grow. You should be patient and slow with any exercise. Lifting is not a race. It's an artistic art. You must ensure your feet are planted on solid ground and that your posture is correct. You should not slouch, or be half-assed.

Lower cable flyes will require the same number and repetitions. Drop the cables completely to the ground. Grab the cold, steel handles. The first one you will need is to face your fingers forward and keep your arms straight at the elbow. Slowly increase the weight. Your fingers should be within a few inches of your forehead. Slowly decrease your weight.

By now, you should be taking a look at yourself in the gym mirrors, and saying, "Wow, I'm pretty damn good." As you begin to look at yourself, you move on to the man zone.

We are now at dumbbells. Place a bench on the ground, then recline it to a 45-degree angle. I will usually use the same dumbbell weight for an incline presse, then I will grab a lighter one for a workout set. This is all I know. Listen to yourself and do what you feel is right for your body.

Get the weights down on your knees, grip them tightly, and you can then lift them up. You want to create a mind-muscle connection and get that chest pumping. I am more about power than looks so I keep my elbows in place and squeeze hard. It is important to keep everything in place throughout the whole range of motion. Exercising too often can place a lot of pressure on your shoulder. Trust me, you don't need a jackedup rotator cups when you love lifting.

Now, lower the weights slowly with the weights still high above your head and your elbows almost locked out. They should feel natural to lower, around the area of your nips. Once the weights are at the bottom of your arms, place them parallel to the deck. Next, stop and push them back up until their ends touch. Focus on your chest when pushing the weights back up. Imagine that you are trying to squeeze your man's pecs in for a snapchat selfie.

Continue this exercise for around 8 sets of 12-15 reps. Stop. You don't have to say everything as fast as you possibly can. I just said as many as I can. It's important to keep the basics in mind. Take it slow and steady. This is bodybuilding.

Incline Dumbbell Press

If the machine is not taken, go to the sit down fly. A moderate to good weight is your goal, but nothing too extreme. The handles are to be held in your hands by a firm grip. To catch any fly, I keep my hands open while the handle rests in my palm. This allows for you to target the chest better than pressing the handles hard and having your biceps help. Keep your arms bent and reach for your hands. Some machines require you to use your forearms, instead of your hands. This is the same concept with a slight twist. Another 8 sets, 12-15 reps.

Machine Chest fly (Forearm).

These exercises will get your started. You can also change it up by doing flat dumbbell press or incline bench. Simple pushups are something else I do. Every set, change your hand position so you're targeting different areas. You'll feel the heat if you do at least 5 sets of 30 minutes after your workout.

Dumbbell Fly

You might be reading this thinking, "Well, I wouldn't do that." Let's go to traffic. This is a very basic guide for anyone looking for some help. Barney Style.

Chapter 8: A Work-Out Plan For You

Essentials for Your Personal Program

DIY girls can be a great way for a beginner to bodybuilding. It will allow you to explore the benefits of different exercises as well as how they are integrated into your own program. It will allow you to create your own personal training program.

This section can be helpful if you're not familiar with the basic workouts or need to know more about how to create a training program.

These are the essentials of every weightlifting training program.

Compound Lifts

Compound lifts include exercises that involve two or more muscle group. These are critical for building muscle and losing weight. This rule of thumb states that you should include at least 2 of these exercises in your workouts.

These compound moves are good for building lean muscles and for improving your mobility. These compound motions usually involve a series of fluid movements that keep you agile and fast. Because they raise your heart rate, you can benefit from it being good for your cardiovascular system.

These exercises are more intense than any other lifts because they involve multiple muscle groups. As an example, squats engage all of your leg muscles, back, abdominal, and stomach muscles. Thus, they burn more energy. Compare this to leg press that isolates your quad leg muscles. You will see a significant increase in calories.

Compound Lifts

Squats

Push-up

Dips

Deadlift Bench press

Pull-up

Push press

Lunges

Accessory Lifts or Isolation Lifts

These lifts could be called your "friends" in compound lifting. These lifts can be used to target muscles or muscle groups that are more defined or stronger. There should be no more than two to four of the following exercises per workout. You can adjust this depending upon how much compound lifting your do.

Since they are not as hard as compound lifting, you will find that isolation lifts will dominate your workouts. You can use them to increase the shape of your body. They are great to treat problem or weak spots. This is the place where toning occurs.

Accessory Lifts or Isolation Lifts

Biceps curl

Triceps push-down

Leg curl

Side and front raise Triceps extensions

Calf raise

Leg extension

About Sets, Reps

The most basic exercise for bodybuilding is three to five sets. Each set would include eight to 12 repetitions. For example, a set would consist of twelve bicep curls. That's equivalent to 36 curls total if you do three sets. This is the ideal range to help muscle development.

For beginners, you need to be consistent with your form. It means that the eighth repetition should be identical to your first. If you cannot get to the eighth rep, then you should decrease your weight. If you are just starting to master the movements, it's a good idea for you to start with lighterweights. This will give you the foundations you need and keep you safe. Feeling confident and comfortable is the best way to start adding weight and challenging yourself.

It is common for isolation lifts to have higher reps while lifting lighter weight. While compound lifts typically have fewer reps but lift more weight. Keep in mind that isolation exercises are for building strength while compound exercises help to shape your body.

Rest Periods

The importance of rest is as great as the work itself. They are essential to keep you energized and able complete your workout. While shorter intervals between sets of around 30 seconds will tax your body, they can be used to great advantage if you are training endurance. If you are doing heavy lifting, it can help to rest for a while after each set.

Progression: How to Take Advantage

The system of progress is the secret to great training programs. You will see a difference in your body if you change your workout. Stamina will result if you continue doing the exact same exercises with the exact weights. It is important to challenge yourself to lift more weights and get stronger until you attain the body you desire. Once you're comfortable with your training regimen, it's time to start changing it. There are many ways to increase your training program's effectiveness. This will make you feel better and it will start to show on your body.

Cardio Training

Cardio is the heart of your cardiovascular system and it will help to lift more. A stronger pair if lungs and a strong heart mean a stronger overall body.

Each cardio exercise program has its own pros, and cons. The one that is most suitable for you will be the best. Here are some suggestions for your cardio.

High Intensity Interval Training

This is a highly effective way of burning fat. It is also very straightforward. The only thing you have to do is to exercise. This can be done with cardio equipment as well as your own body weight. It's important to do intense exercise first, then rest for a while and then go back to it. You can start by starting with half an hour of intense work followed by half an hours of rest. This can be repeated fifteen to twenty times. You can eventually learn to work harder and relax less once you're comfortable.

Weight Training

Weights are another option for those who can't stand treadmills or stationary bikes. Reduce the time between sets and exercises when you do regular weight training. It will be easy to notice an increase in heart rate while working out. This means that you burn more calories lifting weights. This can save you time and allow you to avoid boring treadmills.

Low Intensity Stady State

Another common option for women to do cardio is the elliptical machine. It requires you to spend approximately twenty to thirty minutes at fixed cardio machines. This exercise is more intense so you will need to do a longer workout. This is not the best method to lose weight and calories. As they do not have the energy for intense cardio, bodybuilders or athletes resort to this strategy only when they are on low carbohydrates.

Endurance Training

This is a great option if you love running, swimming or biking. The goal is to build athleticism via long runs (swims, rides), and other activities. This can be integrated in your bodybuilding program, by scheduling your cardio on days when you are not planning on doing weight training.

This will allow you to exercise more and lift more weight when you're needed.

Chapter 9: The Right Age to Bodybuild

It doesn't matter how old a woman is, bodybuilding can be done by them regardless. There is a time when your weight training can be started without having any negative effects on your body.

Young teens' bones, muscles, and bones are still growing so it is best to not interfere with their growth by lifting weights or doing resistance workouts. Your muscles and skeleton will be fully developed at 20 years of age, so it's best not to begin serious bodybuilding. There is still much debate as to when it is best to begin bodybuilding.

Many teens continue to lift weights for muscle growth and improved performance in sports. The teenage bodybuilder's program is different from the one for those who are older than 20. It is used lighter weights and the training goal is to improve muscle mass rather than increase performance.

Although bodybuilding is possible at any age over 20, it is much more difficult to do so with a 20-year-old than with a 50-year-old. The body of a 50 year old woman is not as strong as that of a person in their prime. This means that the level and intensity of bodybuilding must change to compensate.

As young as 13 years, a girl's bodies will turn into a man's. A proper diet and exercise will ensure that her body is in its best shape by the time she reaches 20. She can keep her best shape until her 30s. As she gets older, her body begins to age. Her skin will begin sagging and her body shape may change. These are the most common times that women turn to exercising.

Bodybuilding is one of most popular ways for women to slow down their aging process. Women lift weights to build muscle and firm their skin. You also lose fat in the process which can contribute to your body's rapid aging.

Cardiovascular exercises, such as aerobics, are vital for aging women. These help keep the heart and lungs in good condition and increase endurance. These two things aren't sufficient to build a healthy body. Although they will lose fat, they will also leave you with a lot of skin. This is not a good look. The best way for women to get firm skin is to lift weights. Although bodybuilding isn't as effective for women as it is for men, it won't result in a woman looking more masculine or feminine. You can have fun building your body with bodybuilding just like other fitness activities.

Chapter 10: First Lose Pounds

Before you can start bulking up, you have to cut. This means you need to shed those extra pounds. Understanding this, you will find that the best way to lose weight is to eat less. Losing weight is as easy as eating less calories.

Most bodybuilders will cut before they bulk. However, we can't turn fat into muscle.

If there is a net loss, that means you are in a caloric surplus. Every diet from paleo to low-carb is designed to achieve a caloric imbalance.

You diet is the key to losing weight. Secondary factors include how many calories your body is burning and how much you are eating. A 2 mile run will result in about 200 calories. As you can see, this is very tedious. This is why so many people end up overweight. Our logic tells us running for two consecutive miles must have been a ton of work. However, in reality, all that was done was the one-cup of ice cream consumed.

If you really want to lose weight, then you must learn to control your eating habits. There is hope. Here are some strategies:

Strategy One: Counting Calories

This all depends on what type of personality you have. Are you someone who is obsessed about numbers and measurements. If so, calorie count may be right for your needs. Most people find it very hard to believe that we can do this without feeling trapped. Instead of being free, we have constant analysis.

To count calories, it is important to examine the nutritional facts of every item and keep a piece of paper. This is how we see many dieters, especially women who like to eat out often.

This can be problematic:

1: It's inaccurate. Many restaurants don't list the exact amount of calories they serve. We don't have any idea what the chef is up to backstage.

2. It's very tempting for cheaters. It is amazing to me how many times someone has said, "Oh fuckit, I'll just have the ice-cream. YOLO AMI RIGHT LOL!" To pull off this feat you will also need great discipline.

Strategy Two: Meal Preparation

Alternative options are to cut out the need to go to restaurants or shops often and prepare all of your meals in advance.

This takes perseverance as well as discipline. But, I think it's a better bet since you will always know how much of each meal you eat at any given time. This eliminates the temptation of cheating as your only source to food is what you prepared.

Tupperware containers can be a hassle. You will need to keep a cooler on you so you can take it with you everywhere.

Use the following equation by cutters to calculate how much you will need to pack.

Body weight in pounds x 10 = fat reduction calorie consumption

If you're trying to stay within a calorie deficit and have a weight of 250 pounds, this will tell you that you need to multiply 250 by 10.

Strategy 3: Don't wing it but eat smart

I find it very satisfying to divide my food up so that I know exactly what I am consuming. I can't be tempted with those God Knows What chicken nuggets if I'm at work, school, or both. Because I know I have lunch with my in-built cooler, I don't get distracted. It's not always easy, but it keeps me on track. It's also easy to know that I don't put unnecessary junk in my body because I buy my ingredients.

There is however another strategy called EATING SIMPLE.

This is a more complicated strategy and may require you to use the second strategy. It is important to plan your meals well in advance if preparing them yourself. These are some other tips for when you go out to dinner. Here are some important tips

Eat Consistently

It is amazing to know that the ancient Spartans survived by only two meals per day. Sparta called it the "black soup," which consisted of blood, meat shoulders and spices. Some rice or wheat was added for energy. This is what Spartan warriors ate every single day.

You must do the same thing. But you must do it consistently. So if you're preparing meals, make sure to count the calories and figure out what you should eat.

Just think: Protein + Healthy Carb + Something Green. This will help you know what to eat.

Some examples of meals are:

White meat (slab of poultry), broccoli, and Quinoa.

Fried tofu (asparagus, almonds)

Egg white egg omelet, chicken, fried cabbage, almonds

Sliced pork and cabbage, brown rice

These are the next rules, regardless of whether you prefer to cook at home or eat out frequently.

No White Carbs

White carbs contain SUGAR which is also called glucose. Your energy levels will rise if you consume a lot of white carbs. All of this white sugar will also be converted into high caloric foods. All of this is a problem for any dieter. This is why so many West people are not only overweight, they're also likely to have diabetes and other health problems.

Continue to avoid white carbs.

Here are some white carb examples:

- All white loaf

All white cereal

- All white pastas

- All breaded items

- All white potatoes

- All-white flour

- All white

You might be wondering if brown versions are better. Sometimes, yes. The whole wheat bread is slower acting and has less sugar than the white counterpart. However, it's not nearly as great. Legumes (beans) or nuts (such as almonds) can be added to make carbs and proteins even healthier. It's okay to have some brown rice.

Don't Neglect Vegetables

You can ask restaurants to swap out certain items in order to get more vegetables. One example is to swap white rice with a bed of broccoli. Also, don't eat anything but greens when you go out.

Don't Neglect Calories

Beans, legumes, and other legumes are great calorie boosters. You could feel tired if you eat too many calories or go under the suggested amount. Calories are simply units of energy that give us power. (I have to explain what a "calorie" is sometimes to people). It's not an ingredient, where someone adds 1 teaspoon of calories from the jar. It is a unit for energy similar to volts or electricity in food.

Rev Your Metabolism

Next, you need to be CRUCIAL. You can burn weight even when you sleep by improving your metabolism. Your metabolism determines how fast your body processes the food it receives. People with high metabolisms will naturally be very slim. Their bodies burn calories quicker than they store them. High metabolism bodies mean that they are always active and making use of all their energy. Lucky bastards!

If you are not blessed with a fast metabolism, you too can increase it. Below I'll list several methods to achieve this.

Tea: Research has proven that tea can increase metabolism. This includes green coffee. Get a box of green Tea and have it with you all the time.

Water: Water is a great way to speed up your metabolism. It can also help with weight loss.

Cinnamon is one of the many "metabolism-powerhouses" found in Whole Foods' spice aisles. One of them? Cinnamon. Experts predict that you will be cooking more consistently if you add a lot of cinnamon.

Cold Baths. If you're really dedicated, then cold water will speed up your metabolism.

Star athletes and celebrities might take ice baths after meals if they need to lose weight quickly. Do I recommend it? I don't know. It isn't masochistic enough for me!

Don't Chug Calories

Put down your Starbucks latte. It is easy to ruin a diet by drinking habits that are high in calories. The following are examples of things to avoid:

- Don't drink milk

- Avoid excessive beer consumption

- Avoid hot cocoas and sugary coffee drinks

- Don't make your tea with milk or sugar

- You should absolutely not drink soft drinks. There's more to soda than you might realize and it could help you live longer.

- There are no energy drinks. Red Bull etc. contain only calorie-laden chemicals.

Cheat Day

A lot has been said about cheat days in the fitness and building community. According to doctors and dietitians who have studied the subject, the body can become starved if it experiences a prolonged caloric deficit. It believes it must slow down to survive the coming famine. The body will then stop trying to speed up its metabolism, and it will purposely grind everything to a standstill, which results in WEIGHT GHAIN.

Make sure your body is not confused. Once a week, remind it that you're not lost. To make your Monday start a little easier, you can eat whatever you want on Sunday. This means you can go crazy and indulge in ice cream, warm baked cookies, or even a large portion of spaghetti.

This will increase your MORALE. This is a day when you can go out with your friends to eat. Your friends will be able to see that this person isn't completely deprived of normal food.

How long will it take before I start my next set.

Now that you have finished all your reps, it is time to set the barbell aside. You're done with your reps. Now, how long until you pick it up again. There's much to debate here. Experts claim that you should not spend too much time between sets. This can cause hormonal changes, which could lead to an increase in endurance and effectiveness. Some people are able to go wild, catch their breath, and then quickly pick up the bars again for another shot.

This technique, however, has one purpose, which is endurance training. Imagine that you're about entering military bootcamp.

These activities demand muscular endurance, and you don't need to pause. If this is the reason why you are doing your workout, then I recommend you to do your sets that way and don't take too long for recovery.

But if your goal to gain MASS it's better not to rest in-between sets. If you rest, your ability to continue working out will improve without causing fatigue. You will likely finish your entire workout. Use a stopwatch to keep track of your progress and allow you to wait 2-3 minutes before picking up again. Do this after each set.

You're probably wondering what I would do if it were me. I would leave my smartphone in the car and hide it behind the windows so nobody sees. Why? It's tempting to look at memes while you sit between sets. This will make your 2-

minute recovery time into 15 minutes full of fuckery.

This points me to...

How long should I spend at the gym?

8 sets of compound exercises will be performed. Each set will have 6-7 reps. The weight is targeted for muscle loss. I will take 2-3 minutes off between sets. Also, there will be 20 to 30 seconds of tension per rep. This makes it about 20 minutes each time. I'm usually done by the time I finish three exercises in a session if I don't do any mistakes. It's actually an hour, ten minutes. That includes the time I spend in the locker rooms changing into my gym clothes. Optional, you can use the gym shower. This isn't something I like to do, but I will do it if there's a post-gym commitment (like going back to work).

It is important to be efficient with your time. If you spend too long at the gym, chat to people, use your phone, etc., it is possible to end up staying there for two hours.

It's great to work out and go to the gym. However, my goal in lifting weights is to make my muscles stronger and more flexible.

Hopefully this will give you an easier way to allocate your time.

Important Notes

When you're a bodybuilder it is essential that you get at least 8-10 hours sleep each nights. When your body does all of the work, such as recuperating and renewing itself, sleep is what it does best. As you sleep, these torn cells are being rebuilt into newer versions of their self.

Some of these basic functions can not happen smoothly if water is not available. Dehydration causes a slowing of your metabolism, which can lead to reduced capacity to repair damaged cells.

Also, keep your joints lubricated to prevent injury. A dry body can lead to injury. It detoxifies your body and helps you stay fit throughout your training sessions.

How much water should you use? The best thing to do is just to go. Keep a full liter of water handy, fill it up when you can, drink throughout the day, and make sure to keep it filled. Unless you're an obsessive or compulsive water user, you don't need a logbook to track your water consumption.

Drink water even if you're not hungry.

It is possible to get dehydrated if your urine has a dark, or even very pale, color.

It is impossible for you to get hydrated from drinking coffee, soda, or almost any other sugary drink. It's incredible to me how SODA is consumed all day to fuel their bodies. They do not think twice about peeing dark yellow. You end your day with ALCOHOL. Their skin turns puffy, they become sick with a drop of a hat, and combined with smoking, they begin to prematurely age.

You don't have to be like everyone else. You need to be aware of this vital part of your body.

Becoming A Gladiator

This concludes this practical method portion of the book. I have provided all of the information required to make you a success. A lot more fitness books than this one would be a waste. There is no need to continue with your workouts. Your muscles will not be built by lifting books, or clicking on a mouse. Only going to the fitness center and working hard at it will do the trick. Don't feel the need download another fitness manual. Instead of getting closer to your goals you are mentally MASTURBATING and not taking action.

It is possible to immediately apply all the advice. The next book you should read should be called Advice for Bad-asses. It should include a photograph of you at the front. There are always more ways to grow as a person. I will mention this briefly in the next chapter. Bodybuilding is about doing physical actions, not sitting at your laptop and reading.

Mind-blowing, but also very cool.

Chapter 11: Supplements The Five-Color Strategy for Nutrition

Wall Street is covered in gold, thanks to the tens-of-billions of dollars that are invested each year on nutrition, vitamins, and supplements that will make your life better.

All it is, however, is poppycock. Everything comes with a price. The more citizens spend their hard-earned money on useless promises and supposedly new options the more self-deluded, ultimately depressed, they will become. This cycle is repeated ad nauseam. Another supplement will be discovered deep in the Amazon jungles. Yet another big-pharma breakthrough for body-building, lean-control, weight-loss will be made. We all know this as well as the moon and stars - it's the only way that a multibillion dollar industry is built upon our unhappiness with ourselves.

Let's get back to Tess, our friend. According to her, balance is crucial. You can look at your body and ask yourself if you have any fat stored for energy. Would it make sense to add more fat without exercising? First and foremost, we should avoid any food that isn't necessary to our bodies for nutrition. To begin building your body, you can add those non-natural ingredients to the mix.

Now let's supplement the nastiness we've removed and enhance our body-building experiences! You haven't gotten rid of the notion that "supplement" is not available in a single bottle. Good! We now have the ability to supplement our diets and add nutritional supplements after exercise.

Five-Color Strategy - Each day, pick five fruits/vegetables from five different color families! It's that simple. No, candy corn does not qualify! This is how it should be looked at. What fruits and vegetable do you eat every morning? You can write them down. Keep a journal! This journal will serve as your best friend for the remainder of your life. It's not necessary that you write complete sentences each day. Or use Oxford Dictionary words. This journal is perfect for you. It is crucial to the perseverance aspect of your triangle of bodybuilding. Training, nutrition, endurance. Write it down and retain the words. Write it down on the chalkboard. Stick one of these sticky reminders on your computer at work. Although we will be talking about perseverance later in this chapter, I ask that you immediately begin your journal. Here's why.

You will change your Five Color Strategy every day after you've chosen them. That's why this regimen will work. For breakfast, you may have a banana yellow with your oatmeal (grain), and a salad greens with tomato (red), red cabbage (purple). Add some olives, green or black, if desired. For dinner, a poached and skinless chicken breast (protein), is best. For dessert choose a pear (white).

Another possibility: One soft-boiled yolk (protein), one 12-grain organic piece of toast (brown), nonfat (no add sugar) yoghurt [protein] with fresh raspberries(red) for lunch, poached fish (protein) and spinach (green) salads with cold baked squash (yellow), Spanish onion (purple) or red-and -green grapes (red and-green) for dessert

You will enjoy choosing your Five Colors. Perhaps the rest of you and your family will also like to have a go at it.

Boredom can be a major enemy for body builders. You should change your Five

Colors each week (and record it in your Journal!) One week is too long to remember what you ate. Keep your protein intake up to date. You don't have the need to be concerned about added sugars if you aren't eating prepared foods. However, you do need to monitor your salt intake.

Salt as an addictive supplement: salt is deadly because it can increase body weight, fluid retention, or cause an imbalance. Sodium is naturally found in foods. However, some foods contain more sodium than others. Tomatoes have high sodium content while lettuce does not. Global society insists on a supplement that is no longer valid. Salt was used before refrigeration to preserve foods. A block of salt and bread were found on King Ludwig's personal dining table at Neuschwanstein Castle (Bavaria). These were gifts of Russia's Czar and Czarina, and

I asked him what they meant. He explained that the bread was for warmth and personal gestures and the saltblock because salt was just as valuable in those days as gold. We are able to freeze food and cure without salt. Sea salt can be used to flavor your favorite foods. Don't let other chemicals-based supplements (salt substitutes or sugar substitutes) fool you. Change your daily routine. You will feel much less bloating or edema and your salty taste disappears!

Before you begin any body-building activities, always consult a nutritionist. Nearly all nutritionists are free to be found at your doctor or at the college or university. They may have interesting substitutions that could be made for you based on years of data. All insurance policies must now include a provision to cover wellness checks, and often these include nutritionists. They are essential!

We have given up smoking, and we now choose to preventive care for our bodies. This is an integral part of body-building strategies.

Hypoglycemics (like me) need to have some protein every couple of hours to maintain the balanced "Tess" recommended. I have a simple supplement that I use, which is very easy to prepare and extremely helpful after a stressful day. Trader Joe's can be a great source of these powders as well, as are any nutrition outlets like Whole Foods and GNC. These products are very affordable. I can also combine yogurt, fruit juices, and fresh fruits so that I not only get my protein, but also the super-qualities of blueberries strawberries, bananas raspberry, blueberries peaches, mangoes, papayas, and other superfoods like blueberries, strawberry, raspberries. You can make different shakes every day by mixing them. Put everything in a blender. Then, let it sit for a few hours before you take it out.

Supplemental vitamins, and minerals, are both safe and cheap. Chelated vitamin and mineral supplements such as those available at Trader Joe's are safe and inexpensive. They directly enter the cell's mitochondria. We all are unique. We all have different bodies. If your body doesn't have the right nutrients, it will start to emit red lights and sirens. Listen to the body.

Chapter 12: Exercises for the Belly

The belly fat, which is considered the worst and most harmful fat, is undoubtedly the most unhealthy. This chapter explains the different exercises that you can do in order to eliminate belly fat.

Crunch Beat

This will help you to target your lower abdomen.

How to do it

- Lye on your back

- Bend down and lift your calf muscles.

- Now, put your hand behind the head and extend your elbows.

- Don't lift your shoulder from the floor

- Cross your ankles by moving your legs diagonally.

- You should hold this position for 8 second.

- Continue doing this for the next ninety seconds, with a 10-second break after each crunch.

Single Bridge

This will also target your stomach! Two birds, one stone

How to do it

- Now, lay down on your back with your knees bent.

- Keep the arms in your side

- Now extend your left foot towards the ceiling.

- Lift your hips high off the ground. Now, form a line connecting your right and left knees.

- Now, raise your arms and make 8 clockwise rotating motions. Repetition the movements in the reverse direction.

- Next, move the leg to the opposite side and repeat the procedure.

- Repeat this for the remaining 60 seconds.

Victory Lunge

This applies to your entire abdomen as well.

How to do it

- Stand with your feet apart.

- Place your palms inwardly and raise your hands.

- Squat forward with your right knee.

- Bend your knees towards 90 degrees while keeping your left leg straight.

- Lean forward slightly while lowering your arms behind.

- Next, do the same thing with your left knee.

- Continue to do this for 20 times. Move on and switch legs.

Plie Pose

That's right! This is due to the ballet pose.

How to do it

- Stand with your legs straight apart.

- Rotate your feet so that they are at a 45 degree angle

- Squat with your knees elevated above your ankles.

- Move your arms in front. Keep your elbows slightly bent.

- Elevate your body! Keep your left heel on your right forefoot and your arms high above your head.

- Lower yourself into a squat.

- Next, do the same thing with the right foot.

Continue this twenty-times, switching between your feet.

Chapter 13: Additions

There are many products on the marketplace for bodybuilders. All of these supplements are meant to enhance your body's image (by increasing the size of your muscles). Many of these products are designed to help you maximize your potential for success in the gym. Now the question is: Which supplements should you use?

Creatine

Creatine is one the most sought-after bodybuilding supplements. Because it can increase fat-free muscle mass, professional and amateur builders alike use it. Numerous scientific studies have shown the effectiveness creatine supplementation. Additionally, there is a lot of evidence that it works. These supplements can not only increase fat loss but also improve one's anaerobic as well as aerobic performance.

Creatine can be found in red beef and is produced naturally from the amino compounds glycine (methionine), and arginine. The kidneys, liver and pancreas all play a role in creatine production.

Our bodies have almost 60% creatine phosphate (Cp), and 40% free creatine. An adult male can take in up to 2 g of creatine each day. This amount can also be replenished through food (and the body's natural production).

Adenosinetriphosphate (ATP), which is found in our bodies, is what drives the muscles of our body. It is vital to synthesize ATP again using creatine. When a muscle in the body contracts, the bonds that make up the ATP molecule are split that yields the adrenosine-disphosphate (ADP) compound. This exothermic process of bond breaking releases energy that can be used to power muscle contraction.

When the ATP is insufficient, our muscles are unable to contract. Although there are several ways to lower ATP levels in the body you can use creatine phosphate (Cp) as the fastest. Cp, a compound that breaks down to reveal the phosphate component of its molecule, is called a compound. Cp's phosphate molecule bonds to ADP in order to get back ATP. Once the body has exhausted all creatine phosphate, it will look for another way to revive the ATP levels.

Creatine supplementation increases levels of creatine phosphate in the muscle cells. This results in a higher capacity to recover ATP. The creatine pills increase our body's ability, in simple terms, to maintain a consistent power output to our muscles during high intensity exercise. Without the creatine, it is impossible to complete high-intensity training for the desired time.

There are two main phases to taking creatine supplements. The first is the "loading phase", where you add creatine back to your diet. For one week, you'll need to take 20g daily of creatine during this phase. After this phase, the "maintenance period" begins. This is where you decrease your creatine intake to five grams per day.

But, this is just a guideline. The actual amount of creatine your body requires depends on your body mass. Experts advise that you should consume 0.3g per kg of body mass in the "loading" phase. This means that, if you are 90 kg in weight, the formula would be:

90 kg * 0.3% Kilogram = 27 grams daily of creatine!

After the loading phase is completed, you need to multiply your daily weight by 0.03 grams creatine per person in order to be eligible for the maintenance phase. Now, for someone with a body mass of 90kg, the formula is:

90 kg * 0,03g/kilogram = 27.5g of creatine/day

Creatine consumption will increase muscle mass. This is what makes the muscles look fuller. Additionally, creatine will provide the ideal environment for muscle growth. It will make exercises more enjoyable and prevent fatigue caused by repetitive workouts. Creatine should be taken regularly to maximize its effectiveness. This is not the right way to go.

As stated above, creatine can also be necessary to improve the body's aerobic performance. Creatine supplements are known to lower the oxygen cost for activity, according to a study. This is the amount of oxygen consumed during activity. You will experience less stress when you exercise aerobically. This will allow you to work harder, build more muscle and do so effectively.

The safest form of creatine for health is the one that's not prescribed for individuals with renal disease. If you have any questions please consult your physician.

Bodybuilders typically take creatine powder along with a shake. For added flavor, mix the creatine powder in a shake with either soy or skimmed dairy and add a small amount of your favorite fruits. The best way to increase ATP levels and muscle recovery is to drink creatine shakes after a workout.

Glutamine

Bodybuilders often take glutamine. The body naturally makes glutamine. Our bodies hold approximately 60% of glutamine in their skeletal muscles. The liver, stomach (liver, stomach, and brain tissue) make up 40% of our body.

Glutamin makes up approximately 60% of the amino acid in our bodies. The body can produce more of glutamine in normal circumstances. Supplementation is necessary if the body experiences stress (for example, while exercising).

You have too much glutamine in your body when you exercise. This can cause muscle loss, which is bad news for bodybuilders. Amino acids, the building blocks that make up muscle, can cause the loss of muscle. Amino acids in the body aid in nitrogen transportation, which leads to muscle growth.

Glutaamine not only promotes muscle gain, but also aids with healing and prevents sickness. It can also speed up the production growth hormones.

A typical diet would include 3.5-7.5g of glutamine each day. This compound is found in plant or animal proteins. Glutamine supplements have many benefits and most people choose to take them.

Research also shows that 2 - 40 grams of Glutamine per day is the ideal amount, depending on your needs. It's helpful to ease symptoms such as queasiness with 2-3 grams. You should take 2-3 grams of Glutamine after you have completed your workouts in order to increase muscle protein and recover.

Creatine as well as Glutamine can help you get a lean, toned body. Glutamine is also available in powder form. It can be mixed with a shake.

Protein

Protein is the most essential nutrient to bodybuilding. Protein is what builds muscles and keeps them healthy. The best protein combination is one that includes carbohydrates. These carbs provide the body the energy it requires.

While most of the protein you will need comes directly from your diet, it is sufficient for the average person. For bodybuilders, it is important to increase body mass. For this purpose, the body requires more protein. You should consume more protein by taking supplements. It is vital that you only consume as much protein as your body requires.

Whey protein, which has the highest amount of protein available on the market, is the best. Whey protein makes a great post-workout product because it increases muscle recovery. The post-workout period is critical for bodybuilding. It is during this time that there is severe physical strain on the body, which can cause your cells to quickly exhaust its resources. In order to speed up recovery, ensure you have sufficient protein.

Your body will eventually consume the nutrition to compensate for the lack of protein. This causes your body to produce glutamine, which can eventually lead to a decrease in muscle growth. This is why whey is considered to be the most nutritious protein, especially for those following a diet.

However, whey proteins are expensive so be cautious. Whey protein should still be consumed if you are following a restricted diet. Whey Protein is also a good source of energy, especially if you have a low carbohydrate intake.

Take the protein supplements right after you've done your workout. Your protein powder can be combined with other carbohydrate sources such as eggs, icecream or skimmed Milk. For extra flavor, you might add your favorite fruit to your protein shake.

Nitric Oxide

Nitric dioxide is a powerful and effective supplement that could have many benefits for bodybuilders. The nitric-oxid supplement is often used by professionals for a variety of reasons.

The body naturally produces Nitric Oxide. It increases blood vessel internal diameter by causing vasodilation. Vasodilation leads to an increase in blood flow and oxygen transport. It also provides the necessary nutrients for the skeletal muscles.

The supplement improves your ability to lift weights for longer periods of time. It promotes muscle growth, stamina, and speedy muscle recovery. It also boosts energy, which is why some people use it to improve their sex lives.

While exercising, your muscles contract and blood vessels dilate. The muscle pump that we feel is due to the body's natural nitric oxygen. This muscle pump, however is temporary. The nitric oxide only lasts for a few seconds.

The nitricoxid is available as a pill and should be taken in accordance with the manufacturer's directions. You can also buy powdered nicotine oxide from vendors.

Steroids or Growth Hormones

We want to make it clear that growth hormones or steroids are not recommended. They are often used worldwide by bodybuilders. However, these substances can cause more harm than good. This is why they are illegal in many organizations and sports.

Stimulants and growth hormones are known for stimulating the rapid growth of muscles. These steroids can also boost stamina and make you stronger (for short periods of time).

These steroids cannot be condoned in sports because they give athletes an unfair advantage. Professional athletes are routinely tested for these steroids.

It is important, however, to know that steroids can have several benefits. They can be used to treat AIDS, cancer, and other serious diseases. They can help your body fight these illnesses and boost healing. Steroids that are used for performance enhancement can cause serious health issues.

Steroids can cause liver injury and can even cause liver failure. It also increases testosterone production. This can lead to aggressive behaviour, low number of sperm, and decreased libido.

The main reason most bodybuilders take these steroids is to increase water retention. This can lead to anabolic effects that eventually increase muscle growth and recovery. The heart will have to work harder due to the increased water retention. This can cause high blood pressure and even a heart attack.

When the effects are over, the hormone becomes estrogen and causes feminization. This can lead both to an increase in breast size as well as an increase in fatty deposits.

Growth hormones, however, stimulate muscle growth. They are naturally produced within the body. Many bodybuilders use it to speed muscle growth. This can be dangerous.

There is a way to have massive muscles without using harmful or illegal substances, such as artificial growth hormones. Although these substances might increase your body size over time, they can also make you more sickly.

While bodybuilding has traditionally been a man-only sport, the sport has grown to be more appealing to women over time. Today, both genders have a keen interest in the sport.

Chapter 14: Controlling Cravings/Binges

A friend asked me to write a post about this. I thought it was a great idea. But, discipline is more important than ever. It's easy for you to slip. Last time I fell was Aug-Sep 2012, and I was so upset with myself. I finally got my head in order and got back on track. Slipping used be a daily occurrence when I was a teenager. Because I was not able to control my impulses and had no control over my body, it was an everyday occurrence. However, I've made big strides in the past 12 months, with my daughter entering my life and a family to care for. Ok, how can I avoid binging on sweet foods, McDonalds/KFC, or just eating too much?

First of all, the longer you do it, the easier it gets. Then, with some discipline, it becomes easier and easier until it becomes a routine. It becomes easier with time.

A second tip is to know what is good and not good. Many people believe certain foods are better than they actually are. We are all a bit ignorant about the size of things.

Third tip: Prepare your food daily if your family does not have a great cook like your wife, mom, dad, brother/sister or chef. Keep it in Tupperwear in the fridge. Do not eat it. It is important to read labels, learn the basics of nutrition, and even if it is something you already know, make improvements. It's amazing how many tips you can learn from others, such as low-calorie meals that are filling and healthy.

Never go shopping hungry. Do not go shopping hungry, no matter whether you're at the grocery or local paper. You'd be shocked at the products you find if you don't eat.

Consider adding a pint cold water to every meal. This will slow down digestion and give you a longer feeling of fullness. Take a big glass of water if hunger strikes.

Do not eat too many fats if you're a large eater. Moderate use of Ephedrine with caffeine to help fat removal or to suppress hunger during leaning out phases to help you adjust. Long-term use of drugs that kill appetite is not recommended.

Anadrol may also be helpful in reducing hunger. However I have found that it can be canceled when combined with Tren and EQ. Anadrol with Masteron combined with some Eph is great for helping me feel full sooner. I've used it this year successfully to switch from large meals to leaning and getting into the right mindset before I put my Tren in again. Tren can cause people to be lazy in managing their diet as they can get away with more. However, if Tren is used with some eph, you will feel much better. Slowly digesting proteins, such as cottage cheeses, milk and eggs, are great before bed. Personally, however, I like 100g of musselsi before bed. I sometimes wake up hungry around 4-5 am and have a banana if that doesn't work. But carbs before bed, as long you don't go crazy, are acceptable if you don't overdo it.

Avoid eating out with friends that don't exercise or have poor eating habits. While I am not saying you should avoid eating out, it is important to remember that if you go out with friends who aren't trained or have bad eating habits, you don't want them to be taking your weight off.

Avoid excessive alcohol. I'm not talking about a glass of wine or beer with a meal.

But I am referring to the fact that you don't want to get so drunk or tipsy that you end up eating a pizza and kebab all the way home. Don't drink alcohol if you don't feel like drinking a beer. Too far away from your thoughts.

When you cheat, beat yourself up. If you allow yourself to get complacent and dwell on it, it will continue until you feel guilty.

If possible, you should avoid watching cooking programs, cooking books, or the smells of foods. If Jamie Oliver is on the TV or I smell my missus baking cakes, I begin to think about food and get hungry. If you need some morale, check out programs about obese people.

While some people have more self control than others but most people learn more as they go. If you're like me - you love your food - this is a tough lesson. However, eventually you will feel satisfied with how you have learned self control.

Chapter 15: Vegan Food Substitution Guide

Your favorite comfort foods and recipes can still be enjoyed vegan. Many companies are making vegan versions of popular foods thanks to rising veganism. They are continuously improving their products and making vegan living easy!

Cheese

It doesn't matter what brand you choose, it is important to check the label. You can use vegan cheeses in the same ways as dairy cheese, such as Swiss and sliced parmesan. Salt and herbs may be used to spice up faux cheesese if they are not to your taste.

Honey

While debates surround ethical honey usage in vegan communities, it cannot be denied that the bee population continues to decline. It is possible to help them by not taking their food away. A bee makes honey to provide for its survival. There are many options to replace honey like maple syrup, date paste, or agave netar. These alternatives are superior because of their sweetness, as well as the health benefits they offer.

Milk

Milk is perhaps the easiest food that can be substituted. There are more vegan alternatives to regular milk than regular. They include rice, almond and oatmilk. You can make butternut-milk by mixing 1 tbsp. of vinegar into a measuring jar.

Eggs

Tofu is a good alternative to scrambled white eggs. You can either make it by following a recipe on the internet or buy a ready-made tofu scrambler. This allows you to combine the tofu with other ingredients while you cook. If you eat a lot of protein, this could be a staple part of your daily meal plan.

Meat

Finally, the meat substitutes are probably the most important staple for vegan foods. Any meat-based food can be easily made vegan. Even though it can be tedious because you'll be creating a new recipe from scratch, the health- and ethical benefits are well worth it. Toffuti, Boca Burger and Morningstar offer veganized versions to all of your favorite dishes.

As you can see veganizing any dish is simple once you are comfortable with the substitutes. Additionally, it can be therapeutic and satisfying to cook and prepare your own food. Add in the numerous health, ethical and environment benefits veganism offers and it will be no drag at all!

If you are just beginning to experiment with vegan food preparations, finding veganized versions of animal products can be difficult. However, it can be exciting to switch up your traditional eating habits and receive amazing health benefits. A quick trip to your local supermarket will take you to the right place where you'll find all the vegan substitutes.

Best Foods To Build Vegan Muscle

Here is a summary listing of the best plant-based foods to help vegan bodybuilders. We also provide information about their specific macronutrients. By using these nutritional data, you can create a healthy diet for plant-based bodybuilding that will suit your needs, whether it's getting lean or mass building, or just controlling your diet.

Fruits (per Ounce, 28g)

Food Calories Protein(g) Carbohydrates(g) Fat(g)

Apricots 502.0 12 0.3

Apple 72 trace 19

Avocado (1/4) 80 1.0 4.0 7.0

Banana 105 1.0 30 0.2

Cantaloupe 9.4

Grape Juice (100ml), 45.2.59 19 0.08

Grapes 20: 0.1 5.4 0.08

Mango 18 0.1 4.7 1

Melon Honeydew 10 0.1 5.4 0.2

Orange Juice 44.8% 26.1%

Orange 69 1.0 18. 0.21

Pineapple 13.3 1.0 18 0.3

Papaya 10.9 0.1 2.9 0.4

Pear96 1.0 26.0.4

Plum 30 700 8.0 0.2

Peach 38 1.0 9.0 0.4

Raspberries 14.3-0.4 3.3.0.8

Raisins 86.3 0.7 23 0.2

Strawberries 9.1 0.1 2.2 0.3

Watermelon 8.5 0.1 2.5 0.3

Vegetables (per ounce. 28g)

Food Calories Protein(g) Carbohydrates(g) Fat(g)

Asparagus 16 2.03.0 0.24

Broccoli 7.7

Beats 2.35 0.8 2.8 0.2

Butternut squash 11.5 0.3 3.0 0.1

Carrot 30, 1.0 7 0,1

Cabbage 6.8 0.4 1.6 0

Cauliflower 7.0 0.5 2.0 1.66

Courgette 5.0 0.4 0.9 0.6

Garlic 5.0.0.2 1.0

Green peas 24.1.6.4.3.0.6

Kale 6.5 0.6 1.5 0.2

Mushrooms, 6.0 0.8.0.8 0.1

Onion 11.5 3 2.8 0.1

Potato 161 4.0 37 0.2

Pepper 5.6 0.2 1.3 0.2

Pumpkin 5.6 0.0.2 1.2 0.1

Potato 24 0.0 6.0 0.0

Romaine lettuce 6.2 0.6 1.2 0.3

Sweet potato 103 2.0 24 0.1

Spinach 7.0 1.0 1.0 0.1

Tomato juice 16 0.8 4.0 0.1

Tomato 33 2.0 7.0 0.2

Legumes (per ounce, 28g)

Food Calories Protein(g) Carbohydrates(g) Fat(g)

Black Beans 36.8 2.3 6.5 1.7

Lima Beans 33.8 2.0 6.1 0.5

Kidney beans 34 2.4 8.0 1.5

Lentils 32 2.5.5.6.0.3

Tofu 45 (4.9 1.1 2.5)

Split Beans 32.4 2.2 5.8 2.3

Nuts Seeds or Oils (per ounce, 28g)

Food Calories Protein(g) Carbohydrates(g) Fat(g)

Almond Butter 101 2.5 3.5% 9.5

Almonds, 183 6.7.6.7 15.6

Flaxseeds (1 teaspoon) 59.2.3.4.0

Olive Oil (1 Tablespoon) 1190.0 0.0 14.

Peanuts 186 7.8.6.7.15.6

Peanut butter 96 4.0 3.0 8.5

Walnuts 207: 4.5 4.5 21.2

Breads, Pastas, and Grains. (per ounce, 28g)

Food Calories Protein,

Carbo

hydrates(g) Fat,

(g)

Barley, pearl 33.7 7 7.7 7.7 0.1

Bagel, plain 190 7 37 1

Brown Rice 31.1.0.7 6.4.0.2

Bran Muffin (1 small) 178 5 32 5

Oatmeal 17.2 7.3 3.0 0.2

Couscous 38.1 1 6.4 1.

Macaroni (wholewheat), 39.3 14 8 0.2

Crumpets 134 4 26 1

Flour, tortilla 146 4 25 3

Spaghetti, wholewheat

Corn, tortilla (1) 58 2 12 1

Sourdough Bread Bread 88 3.0 7.0 1.0

Rye bread (1 slice), 83.0 16 2.0

White rice 31.0.6 6.8.0.2

Wholegrain Cereal 85 2.0 21.4 0.9

Be mindful of what you eat and how you prepare it. This will make you more efficient at the gym, which will in turn improve your performance, and ultimately, improve your health.

Chapter 16: Some Basic Exercises

Chest Exercises:

Barbell chest press:

Starting position

Keep the bar steady with a common grip. The elbow should be at approximately 90° and the arm should be parallel to ground.

If you are lying on your stomach, make sure that your eyes are in line with a barbell.

Make sure you contact 5 points (left foot and right foot, lower and upper backs, backs of head, and backs of heads) while keeping your natural arch in the back

Eccentric phase

Straighten the lift bar

Bend elbow and lower the bar until your upper arm meets the ground.

126

Concentric phase

Return the arms to their starting position. Straighten the arms by extending the arms straightening the arms but not locking them out.

Dumbbell bench press:

Start position

You can sit on a bench and rest your dumbbell on your lower leg.

Set the weight at shoulder level and then lie back.

Place dumbbells at your sides, with elbows aligned at 90 degrees. Position your upper arm parallel and the bottom of the dumbbells.

Concentric phase

To extend arms, press dumbbell with elbows toward side.

Eccentric phase

Lower weight from the sides of the upper chest until the upper arms are parallel on to floor

Dumbbell Incline Bench Press:

Start position

Place your dumbbells on your lower leg and rest on an inclined bench.

Set the weight at shoulder level and then lie back.

Place dumbbells to your sides, with elbows at approximately 90° angle. Position upper arm parallel and lower arm parallel to the flooring.

Phase of concentration:

To extend arms, press dumbbell with elbows toward side.

Eccentric phase

Lower your upper chest and lower weight on the sides until your upper arms meet the floor.

Side note: Dumbbells should follow an arch pattern. Above the elbow, it should cross over the chest at the bottom.

Shoulder exercises

Dumbbell shoulder pressing:

Start position

Keep your feet planted on the floor and bend your knees to 90 degrees.

The back should have a natural arch

Spread your arms and elbows outwards, keeping your elbows in line with the floor.

Phase of concentration:

Press the arms over the head and raise them until they reach the shoulders.

You can raise your shoulder blades by rotating them upward. However, you must maintain a straight spine.

Don't forget your elbows

Eccentric phase

Proper posture and weight reduction are key to lowering your starting weight

Dumbbell shoulder raise (Seated. Lateral).

Starting position

Place your feet on firm ground.

Dumbbell should be pointed towards the outer end of the upper limb, with palm facing inward

Elbows at about 90 degrees

Concentric phase

While lifting dumbbells, you should abduct your shoulder and keep a 90 degree angle to the elbow.

Lift dumbbells up until elbow and dumbbell are parallel to each other.

Eccentric phase

For a starting position, lower your weight

Dumbbell front shoulder raising

Starting position

Grab dumbbells both hands. Place dumbbells in each hand on the front legs of upper legs.

Phase concentratic:

Prop up dumbbells and raise them upward until the upper arms are slightly higher than horizontal.

Eccentric phase

For a starting position, lower your weight

Side note

You can raise both arms simultaneously, alternately, or raise them one after another

If you're standing, ensure that your knees are bent at the knees to alleviate pressure from your lower spine.

Back exercises "latissimus dorsi"

Cable pull down

Starting position

Make sure to grab the cable bars with a broad grip.

Under pad, knees should be secure and there should be some lean back (between 15 and 45 degrees).

Concentric phase

Push the bar toward your chest until your arms reach the ground.

You can pull your scapula together to create a natural arch at the bottom of your back.

Keep your scapula in a down position and do not press it.

Your elbows should point towards the ground.

Eccentric phase

Reposition the arm slowly back to its starting position. Keep tension on the dorsi latissimus.

Once the original degree is established, the hip angle should not change.

Cable row at the seated position

Start position

Put your feet against the machine with your knees bent.

Relax your back slightly, and try to keep your arch in the lower back.

As you hold the handles, make sure your wrists and elbows are not bent while holding them.

Concentric phase

With your arms slightly bent and your shoulder slightly retracted, you can pull the shoulder blades to the side.

To make sure your elbows don't touch the shoulders, pull your arms back so that they are close to your side.

Eccentric phase

Slowly return the arms to their original position.

Biceps exercises:

Barbell Biceps curl

Starting position

Grasp barbell, with common supinated grip "palm faced up"

Stand straight and maintain neutral spine. Your knees should be slightly bent. Your scapulae ("shoulders blade") should be pulled out and depressed.

Concentric phase

To make sure the elbows are fully flexed, lift the barbell so the barbell is directly in front of the chest.

Eccentric phase

Lower the barbell so that your elbows are slightly bent.

Dumbbell biceps curl (seated) with palms facing down

Start position

Place your feet flat on ground.

Grab dumbbells with pronated grip. Keep them at your side, with your palms facing in.

Place your feet on the ground and sit straight.

Concentric phase

While slowly turning the palms up, raise the dumbbells "Suppinating" the wrist

When the dumbbells are lifted to their maximum height, the weight will be directly in front.

Eccentric phase

So that your palms face inward, reduce the weight.

Chapter 17: Eating well

You can make a significant difference in your ability to achieve your goals and build muscle.

Most people don't pay enough focus on the foods they eat when trying transform their bodies. But food is important and should not be overlooked when you are trying to transform your body.

We'll give you suggestions, tips and recipes to help get the results you want. This book is intended for women who wish to create a body-building and strength program. Further, the primary focus of this book is on the diet aspects and requirements necessary to build strength and muscle. The book also includes tips, ideas, and suggestions to help you get moving quickly once you start your physical exercise phase.

We all know we need to eat each day to keep our bodies healthy and happy.

healthy. We need to make sure that the foods we eat provide the nutrients and calories that we require. Calories is a small amount of energy that your body uses for powering organs such your heart, lungs. digestion and kidneys.

It's not enough to count calories. Knowing which calories will give you the best results is equally important. You want calories that give you the greatest benefits when you do your strength and exercise.

Diverse nutrients are essential for energy and performance during training and exercise. Daily intake should include a higher percentage of nutrient rich foods.

Our goal is for you to be healthier, gain muscle mass and become more powerful. The right food groups can help you lose the excess fat on your thighs, buttocks, and stomach.

Carbohydrates, protein, and fats are the three food groups that you need to fuel your body. Here are some tips for your health and muscle-building program. Here are daily recipes that will include carbohydrates, protein, or fats.

It is important to make an appointment to your doctor to determine whether you are physically able to take part in a strength or body building program. Also, get your blood pressure and heart beat measured.

Here are some ways you can improve your home. Then, every day, take a look at your weight.

Next, measure your waist. Get up straight.

All the recipes you will see are intended to build muscle, and nourish your body with nutrients that will make you healthier. You may even be able lose weight. It is possible to reach your goals faster than you think if you just follow the guidelines.

It is important to identify the most important parts of your body and decide what you want to do about it. First, establish your goals for the outcome you desire. Then move on. This book is for women looking to build muscle and increase strength. These tips, recipes and exercises are appropriate for your gender.

Let's talk about nutritious foods that help build strength and muscle. Here are some ways to get the results that you desire.

Protein

A body builder requires a lot of proteins in order to sustain their muscle-building program. Proteins enable the body to create, replace, and repair muscle tissue.

This means that proteins are the core of our body's structures.

Because of its role in building muscle, body builders need to know about nitrogen balance. How fast and how much muscle we can build is determined by the nitrogen intake and its release.

The idea is that if you consume more nitrogen than your body needs, your body will use muscle to get it.

This is known as negative Nitrogen balance, and you should avoid it. When this happens, your body begins to break down muscle and enters a catabolic status.

Catabolic status refers to the condition in which compounds have been broken down into energy that can be used to power your biological processes. This is a state where your body wants to grow muscles.

We know that for a strength and bulk builder of 125lb, you must eat the same amount of calories. But, to build muscle, you will need 1 1/2 more calories.

Fats

You will need fats in order to get your energy. To build muscle, fat can be combined to glucose.

Keep in mind to avoid bad fats. They can raise your cholesterol levels, and could lead to heart disease.

Saturated oils are found in animal product such as meats, seafood, milk products like cheese and milk, as well egg yolks. Limit the amount that you eat every day. Eat healthier snacks like fruits, vegetables, nuts and less meat. Dairy products, such as dairy products, are more easily stored than fats so you should be careful about how much you consume.

This type of fat should not be used for bodybuilding or strength training. These trans-fats often contain toxic chemicals and additives that can make your body sick. They can affect you over time or quickly.

This kind of fat is most commonly found in commercially processed food. This type of fat allows most preserved foods stay fresher longer. Trans fats can also have adverse effects on your body's overall health. They are linked with heart disease, stroke, and diabetes.

Trans-fats are everywhere. You should always read the ingredients before buying any pre-packaged snacks or meals from any store. Make smart choices for your health to promote, preserve and renew it.

Unsaturated Fats

Next, we will address unsaturated fatty acids which are easier for the body. Many of these can be used to dissolve stored fat tissue. They can be found in fruits like avocados, nuts, and other foods.

Unsaturated fats can be found in liquid form and should therefore be used for cooking. Canola oil and olive oil are excellent choices, as they won't keep fat in your body. They also protect your cardiovascular system and lower your bad cholesterol.

Omega 3 Fatty Acids, the best form of unsaturated fatty fat, should be included into your daily diet. These fats are effective in combating conditions like depression and fatigue as well as joint pain and Type 2 diabetes. These fats have a significant role in protecting our organs and maintaining healthy hair.

Good fats play a crucial role in your body, and can help you build strength. Do not overdo fats. They can cause problems for your overall health. Here are some ideas for healthy eating.

Try nibbling on brazil nuts and walnuts, instead of chips or candy.

Olive oil is an excellent choice when making a salad or cooking with it.

Bake with nuts and seed instead of chocolate and candies.

Sandwiches can be made with tuna or avocados instead of pre-prepared luncheon meals. Fish should be eaten at least 3x a week to increase your Omega-3 intake. Eliminate fast food, trans-fats, and other unhealthy foods from your diet.

If you want to start a strength and body-building program, you need to be careful about what you eat.

The drink of alcohol has no calories so it will not help with your body building efforts. In fact, alcohol can slow down your metabolism and make it more difficult for your body process the foods that you eat.

Here are some other things that alcohol can do to your body. Did you realize that one vodka shot contains 100 calories? Did you realize that alcohol consumption can lead to muscle cell loss?

Did you realize that alcohol can make your body deficient in protein? Finally, alcohol consumption has been shown to prevent absorption and contraction of nutrients, which are essential for muscle relaxation, contraction, and growth. This includes calcium, phosphorus as well as iron and potassium.

These tips, recommendations and recipes will help shape your strength program and bodybuilding plan.

TIP: Before you begin working out, eat at most 1 hour before your scheduled start time. Carbohydrates make up the majority of your body's glucose. Glucose (a simple carb) is stored as glycogen in your muscles. Glycogen can be described as the main form energy that is stored within muscles.

TIP: 2 When you first start a bodybuilding programme, carbohydrates should make up the bulk your daily caloric intake. Eat more complex complex carbs like sweet potatoes, potatoes and whole grain breads.

TIP: Three Remember that slow-burning carbohydrates promote steady blood sugar levels. This can offset fatigue and promote insulin's release, which is the main anabolic hormonal hormone in the body.

TIP 4 Determine the daily intake of carbs for your body. To determine how many carbs your body needs daily, multiply your weight by 2 and divide it by your body mass.

TIP:5 The Anabolic condition is a physiological state in which energy is required to produce growth and maintenance within the tissues of the human body.

TIP: 6 Consuming sufficient fiber will make your muscles more sensitive to anabolism. This will promote muscle growth and help to create more muscle glycogen.

TIP 7: In order to trigger a steady release insulin that will cause anabolic or muscle building effect, divide your carb meals up into six portions. This will allow for steady insulin production throughout the day.

TIP: 8 Avoid eating too many carbs in a single sitting. It will lead to fat-storing enzymes being activated and eventually, you will start to lose your lean appearance.

TIP: 9 Consuming high carb meals prior to your workouts or training session will lower the chances of fat being stored. Carbohydrates will replenish low glycogen levels before they are able to stimulate fat storage. Here, consume approximately 25% of your daily carbs.

TIP: Ten after sleep, blood sugar and muscles glycogen levels are low. To be able to work out and feel satisfied, you should eat carbs at the beginning of the day.

TIP: 11 Consume carbs as soon as you can, before your body starts to store them as fat.

TIP: 12 If you overuse proteins, it can turn into fat.

TIP: 13 Protein is another vital nutrient every bodybuilder needs. Protein building blocks, amino acids should be part of your daily diet.

TIP:14: Protein is required to grow, heal, and replace tissue. Proteins are a building block for the body, which is why they are so important for those who build strength and bodybuilders.

TIP: 15 - Know your nitrogen level or you could have muscle breakdown. If you lose more of your nitrogen than you take in, this can lead to muscle breakdown. You'll also experience anabolic and muscle building effects if you get more nitrogen.

TIP 16 Avoid negative nitrogen balance. This is when you consume more protein than you take in.

TIP 17: A typical 125-pound bodybuilder will need 125 grams protein. This would correspond to the person's body weight. These protein sources would include meat, fish, or eggs.

TIP 18 Drink plenty of fluids throughout the day before you begin your training. You can build muscle mass by drinking eight to ten glass of water each day.

TIP: 19. Avoid caffeine. This can lead to your body becoming hydrated.

TIP: 20. You will need to drink more water if your supplement plan is to be used in your bodybuilding program. The supplement pulls more water into your cells, creating anabolic effects.

TIP: 21 Allow yourself one week to enjoy whatever food you want. But don't go crazy. You can then return to your strength-building and body-building program.

TIP 22 - Take it easy when you are adjusting to this diet. Give yourself enough time to get used. You will start to crave the foods that you loved once you get used to it.

TIP 23: Try to avoid excessive alcohol consumption while you work out and try to build muscle.

Are you still confused by all these tips? Just remember to eat healthy carbs, proteins, and foods high in fats. Here are some food suggestions that you will find helpful.

You can follow this list to help you choose the right foods for your body.

Here's some food ideas to help you build your body.

Protein- containing foods (Proteins in Grams)

5 oz steak cooked35

5 oz roasted chicken 43

1 egg 6

1. Cup of milk 8

2 slices swiss cheese

2 slices whole wheat bread

8oz. Boiling broccoli 5

8oz. Beans (legumes) 15

Chapter 18: Carbohydrates

Body building is a process that involves protein, fats, carbohydrates, and energy. You might also want to make carbs your primary source of energy when you are doing a lot of hard work. For those who feel fatigued or more tired, increase your intake of carbs.

Complex Carbohydrates

As with fats, choosing the right type and amount of carbohydrates is crucial for body building. Complex carbs contain long chains of sugars which take longer to digest in the human body. Complex carbs provide more long-lasting energy than regular carbs, which can be useful for both your daily routine and the rest. It can also lower the chances of your body storing excess fat. You can find whole-wheat pasta, brown rice, or whole-wheat loaf among others.

Potatoes

This is a low-complex carbohydrate and best for light exercises. It is enjoyed by many people, not only vegetarians but also non-vegans. It comes in chips or baked form. For more carbs and less calories, however, you might choose to make it with less oil or bake it.

Brown Rice

This is an excellent source of complex carbs for heavy workouts. It's not only rich in carbohydrates but also contains calcium, fibre, and iron. All of them are vital for strengthening bones as well as revitalizing cells.

Rotis

This could be one of your best foods when it comes to body building. This is made up of whole grains which are richer in energy and fiber. This complex carb also contains calcium and other minerals.

It is essential to consume a sufficient amount of carbohydrates for body building. It is possible to store fats if your carbohydrate intake is too high. If you are deficient in carbs, it could lead to fatigue. It is best to gauge your fitness level by evaluating when you will do heavy and light workouts. That will help you use your carbs more efficiently and effectively.

Chapter 19: The Natural's Way To Get Ripped

This title includes 2 routines. The first one is for the inexperienced/beginners and the second one is for the experienced.

(Sets x Reps)

Inexperienced Routine -- 4 times per Week

Muscle groups work per week

Chest 2

Arms 1

Back 2

Shoulders 1

Legs 1

Core 1

Monday - Chest or arms

Bench press 5x5

5x5 bench press incline

Bicep curls 5x5

Dips: 4 sets in as many as you want.

Do 4 sets of diamond push-ups.

Tuesday-Back and shoulders

Military press 5x5

Deadlift 5x5

Bent over barbell rows 5x5

Pull ups -- 4 sets of as much as you can.

Wednesday- Off day

Thursday - Legs and core

Squats 5x5

Jump squats: 4 sets of jump squats.

Crunches – As many sets as you can.

Friday - Chest or back

5x5 bench press inline

Deadlift 5x5

Dips: 4 sets in as many as possible

Pull ups -- 4 sets of as many or as few as you can.

Saturday- Off day

Sunday- Off day

Experienced Routine 5 times a week

Muscle groups work per week

Chest 2

Arms 2

Back 2

Shoulders 2

Legs 1

Core 1

Monday- Chest or arms

Bench   press
1x5,1x4,1x3,1x3,1x2,1x1,1x1,1x1

One-handed   inline   bench   press
1x5,1x4,1x3,1x3,1x2,1x1,1x1,1x1

Bicep curls 5x5

Dips: 4 sets in as many as you want.

Do 4 sets of diamond push-ups.

Tuesday - Back & shoulders

Military   press
1x5,1x4,1x3,1x3,1x2,1x1,1x1,1x1

Deadlift 1x5, 0x4, 0x3, 0x3, 0x2, 0x2, 0x1, 0x1, 0x1

Bent over barbell rows 5x5

Pull ups -- 4 sets of as many or as few as you can.

Wednesday- Off day

Thursday- Legs, core

Squats 1x5, 1x4, 1x3, 1x2, 1x1, 1x1, 1x1

Jump squats: 4 sets of jump squats.

Leg raises- 4-sets of as many sets as you can.

Friday - Chest & arms

Bench press 1x5, 2x4, 1x3, 3x3, 4x3, 1x2, and 1x2, 1x1, 1, 1x1

Inline bench press 1x5,1x4,1x3,1x3,1x2,1x1,1x1,1x1

Bicep curls 5x5

Dips: 4 sets in as many as you want.

Do 4 sets of diamond push-ups.

Saturday- Shoulders and back

Military press 1x5, (1x4, 1x3, (1x3), 1x2, (1x2, 1x1) 1x1, 1x1

Deadlift 1x5, 2x4, 1x3, 3x3, 4x3, 5x2, 1x2, and 1x1

Bent over barbell rows 5x5

Pull ups -- 4 sets of as many or as few as you like.

Sunday- Off day

Chapter 20: Understanding Muscle Groups, Exercises

You can't lift weights if you don't pay attention to it. Athletes, trainers, and anyone who works with athletes should be familiar with each muscle's functions to ensure that proper training can take place. The key to reaching your bodybuilding goals is muscle knowledge.

So, let's start. There are two types you can work on when it comes to muscles: the upper and lower.

Lower Body Muscles Upper Body Muscles

Glutes Shoulders

(Deltoids/traps)

Quads Back

(Lats - Middle back, lower back and lower back)

Hamstrings Arms

164

(Biceps, triceps,and forearms

Calves Chest

(Major, minor and combined pectorals

Abdomen Muscles

Upper Body Muscles

1. Shoulders

The muscles above the shoulder called deltoids and are also known by the name deltoids. Anterior, middle, or posterior deltoids are all found under this muscle group. These muscles aid in rotation, abduction, flexing and abduction.

Exercises

Dumbbell Shoulder Press

Side Dumbbell Raise

Dumbbell Front Rise

Bent-Over Rear Rise

Push-Ups (Best for delts, abs, pecs, triceps)

2. Back

The back muscle category includes traps, middle and lower backs.

Lower Back-Keeps the spine stable and core muscles strong.

Lats -- Keep your elbow in line and help to pull the back down and arms down.

Middle Back – Also called rhomboids or stomoids, stabilize the shoulders and keep them together.

Traps-The deltoids are linked with Traps muscles or trapezius muscles. These muscles retract and rotate shoulder blades to support arm weight.

Exercises

Pull-ups

(Best for all back Muscles)

Deadlift

(all back muscles; chest, hips. hamstrings. quadriceps. abs. biceps. legs. hips. and abs).

Cable Row Two-Seat

(All back muscles. biceps. triceps).

T-bar

(middle back, biceps & shoulders)

Dumbbell Rows with One Arm

(lats.traps.and the biceps).

Dumbbell Shrugs

Lateral Pull Down

(lats, biceps, shoulders)

Pull-down grip

(lats. biceps. and shoulders).

3. Chest

These are the major and small pectoralis. These muscles enable you pull your arms backwards and forwards. Several exercises for the chest have been mentioned in previous tables. Here are the other ones.

Exercises

Barbell Bench Press

Dumbbell Bench Press

Dumbbell Flyes

Pullover for Straight-Arm Dumbbells

4. Arms

There are three kinds of arm muscles: forearms, triceps, or biceps. They increase the angle of your joint and extend the arm. Flexors help in flexing the joint and decrease its angle.

Biceps Exercises

Hammer

Barbell Curl

Preacher Curl

Concentration Curl

Cable Curls

Triceps Exercises

Bench Dips

Extensions for the Triceps Lying Muscles

Triceps Cable Extension

Overhead Cable Extension

Close-grip Bench Press

Forearms Exercise

Reverse Barbell Curls

5. Abdominal Muscles

People go to the gym to work out their abs. They are the section of muscle that attracts most attention. To have rock-hard abs you will need to exercise regularly. They are one among the most important muscles, as they support the entire body. They can be classified into transverse abdominal (internal oblique), internal oblique (external) and rectus abdomens.

The transverse abdominals, which support body posture and spine, have the deepest muscle.

The internal ablique supports rotation, bending, support for the spine and helps with spinal support.

The external orblique is located on both ends and aids with rotation, support and bending.

The visible muscles are known by rectus abdominals. They give your body a great six-pack and help you to look good.

Abs Exercises

Before we can discuss the types of exercise you should know, you first need to lose bodyfat so your abs are visible. They're all there. However, the fat that covers them up is what prevents them from being visible. The right diet and regular exercises will ensure you have them.

Crunches in the Abdomen

Leg Raise

Plank

Hanging Leg Raise

6. Lower Body

For some unspecified reason, attention is less given to the lower body. This area needs to be strengthened in order to create an artistic and impressive appearance. Glutes, quadriceps muscles, hamstrings, calves and hamstrings make up the lower body muscles.

Glutes - Move the hip and stabilize the pelvis. They are the largest muscles.

Quadriceps help in flexing hips, legs and hips.

Hamstrings- Help in lower back and hip movement. They also stabilize the pelvis.

Claves are a way to raise the heels.

Lower Body Exercises

Squats

Standing Calf Raises

Seated Calf Raises

Leg Extensions

Lying Leg Curls

Leg Press

Chapter 21: Shoulders

The lateral rise and the military pressing are the two best options to strengthen your shoulder. If you want to achieve a V-shaped athletic body it is important to have strong shoulders. The V-shaped shape of the shoulders is at the top of the body, and the shoulders should be the broadest.

You can shape your shoulders by putting in some effort. To have strong shoulders and rounded shoulders you need to work all parts of your shoulders. The exercises below focus on the shoulders' front and side regions. Back exercises like the row can be used to strengthen the shoulder's back.

MILITARY PRESS

The Military Press, a beautiful exercise, takes us back at the heart of what shoulder power is all about - leveraging stuff low to high.

The barbell, some weight and possibly a pair of hands pads are the essential components of this exercise. With the barbell resting on top of your chest, stand up and lift the barbell into the air. This is your basic movement. It's common for a strong lifter to begin with and to win the first few sets. Then, suddenly, the third or forth set fails. To get the last power, support the lift with your legs. Begin by bending down and doing a slight jump at the same time as the shoulder press.

There are three things you should keep in mind

- Keep your core tight. Maintain a straight back. Tighten your bum. And push your hips a bit forward.

- Stand with the feet shoulder width apart.

- Keep your elbows in line with your hands so that the bar does not fall forward.

LATERAL REISE

This exercise targets the outer side of your shoulders. It will help you to be more broad. If you're just beginning with this exercise, you should start off with lighter weights. If you choose to lift too much weight, it will ruin your exercise. You must utilize momentum from your entire body.

Do not lift weights that are too high or you will have straight arms. You should take your time, go slow and love the odd phase. Time Under Tension is another term that you can look into, but the basic concept is that the muscular must be stressed more often and for the whole movement. Relax and enjoy the stretching, stressing, and relaxation of the "negative" phase as you move down.

There are three things you should keep in mind

- Keep your chest elevated, shoulders back, and face straight ahead.

- Do not fall forward. Keep your upper back round.

- Place your pinky at your highest point when you hold the weights horizontally.

ABS

Those abs. Many guys and girls regard this muscle as the most essential. A great set of abs will make you forget about everything else when your shirt is pulled off. It is difficult for me to pinpoint the reason. I believe that having shredded abdominals is very hard to attain and maintain. Muscle building is one thing.

Low fat is another. Even if you have strong abs and a lot of fat in your stomach, it will make the boundary between your abdominal muscles erode. A common saying states, "A sixpack is achieved in your kitchen."

Splitting the abdominal region into two areas is an easy and efficient way to work your abs. For ab exercises, the main front area and the sides should be covered.

Strong muscles at your stomach are crucial for achieving the ideal six-pack. To train these muscles, contract your abs by moving your breastbone towards your hips. To accelerate your development of your ab muscles, there are three exercises you can do in the next section.

THE WHEEL

The abwheel - a wheel with two levers per side - can be a powerful tool in building strong abs. This is accomplished by sitting on your stomach and grasping the wheel. Then, move your knees towards your knees so that you can roll off your knees. It may seem simple but the task isn't easy.

There are three things you should keep in mind

Keep your spine straight, don't let your stomach drop when you roll outwards.

- Keep straight your wrists. Hands are subject to a lot stress, so don't twist your wrists.

- When you roll out, be sure to look towards the floor. This will make sure that your head is an extension instead of straining your neck.

WEIGHTED HIIT-UPS

Some people can do hundreds or more of sit ups every week. If we want bigger muscles, that is not what our goal. It is important to remember that endurance is important in this context. Our rep range is about 10, so if we fail the 10th rep then we have to add weight to our sit-ups. It is important that you choose a weightplate with which you can perform 10 and only 10 sit ups, while keeping the plate behind your head.

There is no reason why abdominal muscles should be treated differently to the rest. The abdominal muscles don't require a higher rep range. Just go hard.

Conclusion

You have pledged to the Triangle of Body-Building. This includes nutrition, training and perseverance. You have created a sustainable nutritional plan that will benefit you for the long-term. Your toolbox includes supplementary nutrition to help restore balance after stressful situations like long hours at work or intense exercise. You have started a journal that records your nutritional intake, exercise output, and attempts to return your body to equilibrium by bedtime each night.

You don't have to fear being intimidated by Madison Avenue and their Madison Avenue approach for exercise, weight loss, and supplements. This makes you feel insecure and cowered and will increase your desire to buy more.

Instead, consider "Tess" as your alter ego. The entire idea of body-building is contained within one word: balance. You will soon see that your mind is not your friend, but your worst enemy (fried chicken and potatoes with gravy) and your best friend(poached skinless poultry and green beans and mushrooms). Your mind can only be influenced by you. Nobody can fault your ability to bodybuild on your own terms. I can assure you that everyone will notice a healthier, happier and more fit version of yourself. I wish you much energy and success on your journey.

www.ingramcontent.com/pod-product-compliance
Lightning Source LLC
Chambersburg PA
CBHW060327030426
42336CB00011B/1230